GASTRIC BYPASS COOKBOOK

MAIN COURSE

70+ Bariatric-Friendly Chicken, Beef, Fish, Pork, Fish, Salads and Vegetarian recipes for life long eating for Post Weight Loss Surgery Diet

STELLA LAYNE

CONTENT

PORK RECIPES

SEAFOOD RECIPES

SALAD/WRAPS RECIPES

VEGETARIAN RECIPES

COOKING INFO SUMMARY 73

NUTRITION SUMMARY 77

BEEF AND VEGETABLES STIR FRY

 SERVES 8

 PREP TIME 15 MINUTES

 COOK TIME 10 MINUTES

- **1 pound** lean flank steak, cut into strips
- **1/4 cup** fat-free beef broth
- **2 cups** broccoli florets
- **1 cup** sliced bell peppers
- **1 cup** sliced carrot
- **1** green onion, chopped
- **2 cloves** garlic, minced
- **2 tablespoons** low sodium soy sauce
- **1 tablespoon** grated ginger
- **1 teaspoon** stevia

1. In a small bowl, mix beef with soy sauce, stevia and ginger. Set aside to marinate for 10 minutes.

2. Spray a large skillet. Sauté the onion until fragrant. Then add all the vegetables. Cook for 4-5 minutes until vegetables are tender. Remove from the skillet.

3. Add the beef. Reserve the marinade. Cook until the beef is brown. Then return the vegetables, broth and marinade. Stir and cook for 2 minutes.

CALORIES	CARBS	SUGAR	FAT	PROTEIN	SODIUM
99	4.6	1.9	2.6	13.4	337
KCAL	GRAMS	GRAMS	GRAMS	GRAMS	MILLIGRAMS

THAI GROUND BEEF

SERVES
8

PREP TIME
10
MINUTES

COOK TIME
20
MINUTES

1. Spray a large skillet.

2. Sauté the leek until fragrant. Then add garlic and sauté for 1 more minute.

3. Brown the beef.

4. Stir in curry paste and tomato sauce. Simmer for 3-4 minutes or until the liquid is reduced to half.

5. Stir in the coconut milk and seasoning. Bring to a boil. Serve immediately.

- **1 pound** 95/5 lean ground beef
- **2 cloves** garlic, minced
- **1 cup** thinly sliced leek
- **1 cup** no-sugar-added tomato sauce
- **1/2 cup** light coconut milk
- **1 tablespoon** red curry paste
- **1/2 tablespoon** stevia
- **1/2 tablespoon** fish sauce
- **1/2 tablespoon** lime juice
- **1/2 teaspoon** Sriracha sauce (optional)
- **1/4 teaspoon** lime zest
- salt and pepper to taste
- Nonstick Cooking Spray

CALORIES	CARBS	SUGAR	FAT	PROTEIN	SODIUM
106	4.1	2.1	3.9	13.0	270
KCAL	GRAMS	GRAMS	GRAMS	GRAMS	MILLIGRAMS

SPICY BEEF WITH BOK CHOY

 SERVES
8

 PREP TIME
15
MINUTES

 COOK TIME
20
MINUTES

- **1 pound** lean flank steak, cut into strips

- **6 heads** baby Bok Choy, cut in half

- **1 cup** sliced onion

- **2 cloves** garlic, minced

- **2** chili peppers, deseeded and chopped

- **1 tablespoon** grated ginger

- 2 tablespoons fish sauce

- 1/4 teaspoon salt

- 1/4 teaspoon pepper

- Nonstick Cooking Spray

1. In a medium bowl, season the beef with salt and pepper.

2. Sauté the garlic, ginger and chili until fragrant. Add the beef and cook for 3 minutes. Set Aside.

3. Sauté the onion until fragrant.

4. Then add Bok Choy and cook until soft.

5. Add the beef and fish sauce. Mix well and cook for 1 minute.

CALORIES	CARBS	SUGAR	FAT	PROTEIN	SODIUM
114	5.7	1.6	2.6	13.5	469
KCAL	GRAMS	GRAMS	GRAMS	GRAMS	MILLIGRAMS

BEEF STUFFED BELL PEPPER

 SERVES
8

 PREP TIME
5
MINUTES

 COOK TIME
35
MINUTES

1. Preheat the oven to 375°F.

2. Spray a large skillet.

3. Sauté the onion until fragrant. Then add garlic, green onion

4. and green peppers. Sauté for 3 more minutes. Set aside.

5. Brown the beef. Then all ingredients except cheese and tomato sauce. Mix well and cook for another 5 minutes.

6. Fill the bell peppers half the way with the meat mixture. Add cheddar cheese. Then add the remaining meat mixture. Top with tomato sauce and mozzarella cheese.

7. Bake for 20-25 minutes.

- **1 pound** 95/5 lean ground beef
- **4** medium green bell peppers, tops and seeds removed
- **1 cup** canned diced tomatoes
- **1/3 cup** finely chopped onion
- **1/4 cup** finely chopped green onion
- **1/4 cup** fat-free mozzarella cheese
- **1/4 cup** fat-free cheddar cheese
- **1/2 cup** no-sugar-added tomato and pesto sauce
- **2 cloves** garlic, minced
- **2 tablespoons** minced green peppers
- **2 tablespoons** chopped fresh parsley
- **1 1/2 teaspoons** Italian seasoning
- 1 teaspoon salt
- **1/2 teaspoon** ground black pepper
- Nonstick Cooking Spray

CALORIES	CARBS	SUGAR	FAT	PROTEIN	SODIUM
118	7.7	3.6	3.2	15.6	471
KCAL	GRAMS	GRAMS	GRAMS	GRAMS	MILLIGRAMS

SALISBURY STEAK WITH MUSHROOM SAUCE

 SERVES **8**

 PREP TIME **15** MINUTES

 COOK TIME **25** MINUTES

For the Salisbury Steak

- **1 pound** 95/5 lean ground beef
- **1/4 cup** whole wheat bread crumbs
- **1/4 cup** chopped onion
- **2** egg whites, beaten
- **1 teaspoon** salt
- Nonstick Cooking Spray

For the Gravy

- **2 cups** fat-free beef broth
- **1 1/2 cups** sliced onion
- **1 cup** sliced mushrooms
- **2 tablespoons** whole wheat flour
- salt and pepper to taste

1. Combine all ingredients for the steak. Shape into 8 mini patties.

2. Spray a large skillet. Brown the Steak on both sides over medium heat, about 4-5 minutes each side.

3. Add broth, onion and mushroom. Bring to a boil then reduce to low. Cover and simmer for 10 more minutes. Transfer the patties to the serving plate.

4. In a small bowl, combine flour with a few tablespoons of water. Then slowly stir in the mixture. Cook until sauce thickened. Pour the sauce on the steak and serve.

CALORIES	CARBS	SUGAR	FAT	PROTEIN	SODIUM
120	50	0.9	2.9	17.0	566
KCAL	GRAMS	GRAMS	GRAMS	GRAMS	MILLIGRAMS

MEXICAN BEEF SKILLET

 SERVES 8

 PREP TIME 10 MINUTES

 COOK TIME 35 MINUTES

1. In a medium bowl, season the beef with chili powder, salt and paprika.

2. Spray a large skillet, cook the beef for 3 minutes. Set aside.

3. Sauté the garlic, onion and bell peppers until fragrant. Then add mushroom and cook for another 2 minutes.

4. Add broth and salsa. Simmer until the liquid is reduced by half. Stir in beef and cook for 1 minute.

- **1 pound** lean flank steak, cut into strips
- **1 cup** sliced onion
- **1 cup** sliced mushroom
- **1 cup** sliced red bell pepper
- **3/4 cup** fat-free low sodium chicken broth
- **1/2 cup** no-sugar-added salsa
- **2 cloves** garlic, minced
- **2 teaspoons** chili powder
- 1 teaspoon paprika
- 1/2 teaspoon salt
- Nonstick Cooking Spray

CALORIES	CARBS	SUGAR	FAT	PROTEIN	SODIUM
102	4.4	1.9	2.7	13.2	339
KCAL	GRAMS	GRAMS	GRAMS	GRAMS	MILLIGRAMS

INDIAN BEEF CURRY

 SERVES
8

 PREP TIME
10
MINUTES

 COOK TIME
40
MINUTES

- **1 pound** 95/5 lean ground beef
- **1** 14.5-ounce **can** diced tomatoes
- **1 cup** chopped onion
- **1/2 cup** frozen peas, thawed
- **1 cup** fat-free beef broth
- **1/2 cup** fat-free Greek Yogurt
- **2 cloves** garlic, minced
- **2 tablespoons** curry powder
- **1/2 teaspoon** chili paste
- **1/4 teaspoon** ground turmeric
- salt to taste
- **2 tablespoons** chopped fresh Parsley

1. Spray a large skillet.

2. Sauté the onion until fragrant. Then add garlic and sauté for 1 more minute.

3. Brown the beef. Transfer the beef mixture to a bowl.

4. Add turmeric, curry powder and chili paste. Cook for 30 seconds.

5. Slowly stir in broth and tomatoes. Add Peas. Bring to a boil. Simmer for 15 minutes or until the peas soften.

6. Add beef mixture back. Season with salt.

7. Remove from heat. Stir in yogurt and sprinkle with chopped parsley.

CALORIES	CARBS	SUGAR	FAT	PROTEIN	SODIUM
113	6.4	2.9	3.3	15.0	316
KCAL	GRAMS	GRAMS	GRAMS	GRAMS	MILLIGRAMS

SKINNY ENCHILADAS

SERVES
9

PREP TIME
10
MINUTES

COOK TIME
45
MINUTES

1. Preheat the oven to 350°F

2. Spray a large skillet.

3. Sauté the onion until fragrant. Then Brown the beef. Season with salt and pepper.

4. In a large bowl, combine yogurt, soup and half of the cheese.

5. Mix half of the soup mixture with the meat. Divide the meat between tortillas. Roll up and place them in a baking dish. Top with the remaining sauce and cheese.

6. Bake for 30 minutes.

- **1 pound** 95/5 lean ground beef

- **3** low carb tortillas

- **1** 10.5-ounce **can** condensed 98% fat-free cream of chicken soup

- **1/2 cup** chopped green onions

- **1/2 cup** fat-free Greek yogurt

- **1 1/2 cups** fat-free mozzarella cheese

- **1** jalapeno pepper, de-seeded and chopped

- **2 tablespoons** Taco seasoning

- salt and pepper to taste

CALORIES	CARBS	SUGAR	FAT	PROTEIN	SODIUM
149	7.5	0.6	4.3	19.9	495
KCAL	GRAMS	GRAMS	GRAMS	GRAMS	MILLIGRAMS

BEEF CHILI

SERVES
8

PREP TIME
10
MINUTES

COOK TIME
60
MINUTES

- **1 pound** 95/5 lean ground beef

- **1** 15-ounce **can** dark red kidney beans, rinsed and drained

- **1/2 cup** chopped onion

- **1 1/2 cups** no-sugar-added tomato juice

- **1/2 cup** no-sugar-added salsa

- **1 tablespoon** chili powder

- **1/2 tablespoon** garlic powder

- **1/2 teaspoon** ground cumin

- **1/2 teaspoon** paprika

- **1/4 teaspoon** thyme

1. Spray a large skillet.

2. Sauté the onion until fragrant. Then Brown the beef.

3. Add all ingredients and mix well. Bring to a boil. Reduce to low and simmer for 50 minutes. Season with salt and pepper.

CALORIES	CARBS	SUGAR	FAT	PROTEIN	SODIUM
147	14.6	3.7	3.3	15.7	227
KCAL	GRAMS	GRAMS	GRAMS	GRAMS	MILLIGRAMS

CHEESE-STUFFED MEATLOAF

 SERVES
8

 PREP TIME
20
MINUTES

 COOK TIME
60
MINUTES

1. Preheat the oven to 350°F

2. In a large mixing bowl, combine all ingredients except cheese.

3. Spread the meat mixture on a large baking sheet to form a 14"x18" patty.

4. Add the cheese on the meat. Leave out 1-inch on each side.

5. Roll up and Put it in a 10"x15" baking dish.

6. Bake for 1 hour.

- **2 pounds** 95/5 lean ground beef

- **1/2 cup** whole wheat breadcrumbs

- **1/2 cup** chopped onion

- **4** egg whites, beaten

- **2 cups** fat-free shredded cheddar cheese

- **1 1/2 teaspoons** salt

- **1 1/2 teaspoons** ground black pepper

CALORIES	CARBS	SUGAR	FAT	PROTEIN	SODIUM
83	3.6	0.5	1.6	13.7	412
KCAL	GRAMS	GRAMS	GRAMS	GRAMS	MILLIGRAMS

ITALIAN PARMESAN MEATBALLS

 SERVES
8

 PREP TIME
20
MINUTES

 COOK TIME
70
MINUTES

- **1 pound** 95/5 lean ground beef
- **1/4 cup** whole wheat breadcrumbs
- **1/4 cup** fat-free shredded Parmesan Cheese
- **1/4 cup** fat-free shredded mozzarella cheese
- **1 1/4 cups** No-sugar-added tomato and basil sauce
- **1 1/2 tablespoons** Italian Seasoning
- **1/2 teaspoon** salt
- **1/2 teaspoon** ground black pepper
- **2 tablespoons** chopped fresh parsley

1. Preheat the oven to 350°F

2. In a large mixing bowl, combine beef, breadcrumbs, parmesan cheese, 1/4 cup of the tomato sauce and seasoning. Shape into 8 meatballs.

3. Bake for 15 minutes.

4. On an oven-proof skillet, add the remaining sauce and the meatballs. Toss well. Top with the mozzarella cheese and bake to another 15 minutes. Sprinkle with parsley before serving.

CALORIES	CARBS	SUGAR	FAT	PROTEIN	SODIUM
116	6.7	1.9	3.4	14.7	454
KCAL	GRAMS	GRAMS	GRAMS	GRAMS	MILLIGRAMS

CABBAGE AND BEEF BAKE

 SERVES 12

 PREP TIME 15 MINUTES

 COOK TIME 80 MINUTES

1. Preheat the oven to 350°F

2. Spray a large skillet.

3. Sauté the onion and bell peppers until fragrant. Then Brown the beef. Stir in Tomatoes. Season with salt and pepper Set aside.

4. Spray a 9"x13" baking dish. Spread the shredded cabbage evenly. Then spread the meat mixture on top.

5. In a small bowl, mix together tomato sauce and sour cream. Then spread the mixture on the meat.

6. Bake for 1 hour. Then top with cheese and bake for another 20 minutes.

- **1 1/2 pounds** 95/5 lean ground beef

- **6 cups** shredded cabbage

- **1 cup** chopped onion

- **1/2 cup** chopped bell peppers

- 1 14.5-ounce **can** diced tomato

- 1 8-ounce **can** tomato sauce

- **1 cup** fat-free sour cream

- **1/2 cup** fat-free shredded cheddar cheese

- **1/2 cup** fat-free shredded mozzarella cheese

- salt and pepper to taste

CALORIES	CARBS	SUGAR	FAT	PROTEIN	SODIUM
131	9.0	4.8	3.1	17.6	313
KCAL	GRAMS	GRAMS	GRAMS	GRAMS	MILLIGRAMS

BEER BRAISED BEEF

 SERVES
16

 PREP TIME
5
MINUTES

 COOK TIME
3
HOURS

- **2 pounds** lean top round roast

- **2 cans** beer

- **2** large onion, sliced

- **4 cloves** garlic

- **1 teaspoon** salt

- **1 teaspoon** Ground Thyme

- **1/2 teaspoon** Rosemary

- **1/2 teaspoon** ground black pepper

- Nonstick cooking spray

1. Preheat the oven to 275°F

2. Spray a large Dutch oven. Sauté the onion until fragrant. Set aside.

3. Season the meat with salt and pepper. Brown the meat on all side for about 2 minutes per side. Add all ingredients.

4. Cover and cook in the oven for 2 3/4 to 3 hours.

5. Shred the meat with a pair of forks before serving.

CALORIES	CARBS	SUGAR	FAT	PROTEIN	SODIUM
96	3.6	0.8	2.0	13.0	247
KCAL	GRAMS	GRAMS	GRAMS	GRAMS	MILLIGRAMS

SICHUAN SPICY BEEF STEW

 SERVES
16

 PREP TIME
15
MINUTES

 COOK TIME
2
HOURS

1. Blanch the beef in boiling water. Drain and set aside.

2. Spray a wok. Sauté the ginger and garlic until fragrant. Add the chili paste and cook for 30 seconds.

3. Add beef, soy sauce and wine. Stir well and cook for 2 minutes.

4. Transfer to a stock pot. Add the spices and enough water to cover the beef. Bring to a boil and reduce to low. Simmer for 1 hour.

5. Add Radish. Cook for another 30 minutes or until both beef and radish are tender. Garnish with cilantro and serve.

- **2 pounds** lean top round roast, cut into 1 1/2 slices across the grain
- **1 pound** radish, cut into 2-inch pieces
- **5 cloves** garlic, minced
- **4 slices** fresh ginger
- **3 tablespoons** dry white wine
- **2 tablespoons** chopped fresh cilantro
- **1 tablespoon** Sichuan chilli bean paste
- **1 tablespoon** low-sodium soy sauce
- Nonstick Cooking Spray

Spices:

- **4** dried chili
- **2** star anise
- **2** bay leaves
- **1** cinnamon stick
- **1 teaspoon** peppercorn
- **1 teaspoon** fennel seeds

CALORIES	CARBS	SUGAR	FAT	PROTEIN	SODIUM
84	2.4	0.7	2.0	13.0	102
KCAL	GRAMS	GRAMS	GRAMS	GRAMS	MILLIGRAMS

MONGOLIAN BEEF SKEWER

SERVES
8

PREP TIME
8
HOURS

COOK TIME
10
MINUTES

- **1 pound** lean flank steak, cut into strips

- **2 tablespoons** low-sodium soy sauce

- **2 tablespoons** sherry cooking wine

- **1 tablespoon** grated ginger

- **1 tablespoon** minced garlic

- **2 teaspoons** Truvia Nectar

- **1 teaspoon** dried mustard powder

1. In a large resealable bag, add all ingredients. Seal and shake the bag to mix well. Marinate overnight.

2. Preheat the broiler. Thread the meat onto 16 skewers.

3. Broil 3-4 minutes on each side.

CALORIES	CARBS	SUGAR	FAT	PROTEIN	SODIUM
90	1.8	1.0	2.6	12.3	210
KCAL	GRAMS	GRAMS	GRAMS	GRAMS	MILLIGRAMS

CHICKEN AND SUGAR SNAP PEA STIR FRY

 SERVES 8

 PREP TIME 10 MINUTES

 COOK TIME 15 MINUTES

1. Spray a large skillet. Brown the chicken. Add oyster sauce and cook for another minute. Set aside.

2. Sauté green onion and garlic until fragrant. Then add peas and cook until fragrant. Stir in chicken and stir-fry for 30 seconds.

- **1 pound** chicken tender, cut into strips

- **12 ounces** sugar snap peas, , cut into strips

- **1 tablespoon** oyster sauce

- **2 cloves** garlic, minced

- **2** green onions, chopped

- salt and pepper to taste

CALORIES	CARBS	SUGAR	FAT	PROTEIN	SODIUM
59	1.7	0.6	0.3	11.5	118
KCAL	GRAMS	GRAMS	GRAMS	GRAMS	MILLIGRAMS

LEMON THYME CHICKEN

SERVES
8

PREP TIME
15
MINUTES

COOK TIME
20
MINUTES

- **1 pound** chicken tender

- **1/4 cup** lemon juice

- **6 sprigs** fresh thyme, chopped

- **1 tablespoon** lemon zest

- **2 cloves** garlic, minced

- salt and pepper to taste

- Nonstick Cooking Spray

1. In a large bowl, mix the chicken in all other ingredients. Set aside to marinate for 15 minutes.

2. Spray a large skillet. Cook the chicken until cook through, about 4-5 minutes each side

CALORIES	CARBS	SUGAR	FAT	PROTEIN	SODIUM
55	1.0	0.2	0.2	11.3	56
KCAL	GRAMS	GRAMS	GRAMS	GRAMS	MILLIGRAMS

PEPPER-STUFFED CAJUN CHICKEN

 SERVES
8

 PREP TIME
10
MINUTES

 COOK TIME
25
MINUTES

1. Preheat the oven to 350°F.

2. Spray a large skillet.

3. Sauté the onion and bell peppers until fragrant. Season with salt and pepper. Set aside to cool.

4. Slice the chicken breast to form a pocket. Stuff the vegetable and then the cheese.

5. Rub the Cajun seasoning, then salt and pepper on all side of the chicken breast.

6. Bake for 25 minutes

- **4** boneless, skinless chicken breast

- **1 cup** chopped onion

- **1 cup** chopped bell peppers

- **1 cup** fat free cheddar cheese

- **1 tablespoon** Cajun seasoning

- salt and pepper to taste

- Nonstick Cooking Spray

CALORIES	CARBS	SUGAR	FAT	PROTEIN	SODIUM
91	4.0	1.6	0.6	16.3	522
KCAL	GRAMS	GRAMS	GRAMS	GRAMS	MILLIGRAMS

SPINACH FETA CHICKEN ROLL

 SERVES
8

 PREP TIME
10
MINUTES

 COOK TIME
25
MINUTES

- **4** boneless, skinless chicken breast, flattened

- **10 ounces** frozen spinach, thawed and squeeze

- **1/2 cup** fat-free feta cheese

- **1/3 cup** fat-free ricotta cheese

- **1/4 cup** chopped green onion

- **1/4 cup** chopped fresh parsley

- **1 tablespoon** fresh dill

- **2 cloves** garlic

- salt and pepper to taste

1. Preheat the oven to 350°F.

2. Spray a large skillet.

3. Sauté the green onion and garlic until fragrant. Add spinach, parsley and dill. Cool until heated through. Season with salt and pepper.

4. Remove from heat and stir in feta cheese and ricotta cheese.

5. Divide the mixture onto the chicken breast. Roll up. Rub the chicken with salt and pepper.

6. Bake for 25 minutes.

CALORIES	CARBS	SUGAR	FAT	PROTEIN	SODIUM
83	2.1	0.8	0.6	15.0	328
KCAL	GRAMS	GRAMS	GRAMS	GRAMS	MILLIGRAMS

CREAMY SALSA CHICKEN

 SERVES
8

 PREP TIME
5
MINUTES

 COOK TIME
35
MINUTES

1. Preheat the oven to 350°F.

2. Season the chicken with half of the taco seasoning.

3. Brown the chicken in an -oven-proof skillet. Then stir in salsa and the remaining seasoning.

4. Cover and bake for 30 minutes.

5. Shred the chicken and stir in sour cream.

- **1 pound** chicken tender

- **2 cups** salsa

- **1 package** taco seasoning

- **1 cup** fat-free soup cream

- Nonstick Cooking Spray

CALORIES	CARBS	SUGAR	FAT	PROTEIN	SODIUM
92	5.5	4.0	0.2	12.0	296
KCAL	GRAMS	GRAMS	GRAMS	GRAMS	MILLIGRAMS

YOGURT CHICKEN PARMESAN

 SERVES
8

 PREP TIME
10
MINUTES

 COOK TIME
45
MINUTES

- **1 pound** chicken tender

- **1/2 cup** fat-free Greek Yogurt

- **1/2 cup** low-fat mayonnaise

- **1/2 cup** fat-free grated parmesan cheese

- **1/2 teaspoon** salt

- **1/2 teaspoon** ground black pepper

1. Preheat the oven to 375°F.

2. In a medium bowl, mix yogurt, mayonnaise, cheese and seasonings.

3. Line the chicken on a baking tray. Spread the mixture on the chicken breast.

4. Bake for 45 minutes.

CALORIES	CARBS	SUGAR	FAT	PROTEIN	SODIUM
88	5.6	1.4	1.2	13.4	463
KCAL	GRAMS	GRAMS	GRAMS	GRAMS	MILLIGRAMS

HUNGARIAN CHICKEN PAPRIKASH

 SERVES 8

 PREP TIME 10 MINUTES

 COOK TIME 50 MINUTES

1. Season the chicken with salt and pepper. Spray a large skillet. Brown the chicken. Set aside.

2. Sauté the onion until fragrant. Add paprika and cook for 2 minutes. Add broth, tomato and chicken. Bring to a boil then reduce to low. Cover and simmer for 30 minutes.

3. Remove from heat and stir in sour cream before serving.

- **1 pound** chicken tender
- **1 cup** chopped onion
- **2** plum tomatoes, cubed
- **1 cup** fat-free low sodium chicken broth
- **1/4 cup** fat free sour cream
- **1 tablespoon** sweet paprika
- **1 teaspoon** smoked paprika
- salt and pepper to taste

CALORIES	CARBS	SUGAR	FAT	PROTEIN	SODIUM
72	3.7	1.9	0.4	12.2	80
KCAL	GRAMS	GRAMS	GRAMS	GRAMS	MILLIGRAMS

ROSEMARY BRAISED CHICKEN

 SERVES
8

 PREP TIME
5
MINUTES

 COOK TIME
55
MINUTES

- **1 pound** chicken tender

- **1 cup** white wine

- **3 sprigs** fresh rosemary

- **2** bay leave

- **1** lemon, juice only

- salt and pepper to taste

1. Preheat the oven to 375°F.

2. Season the chicken with salt and pepper.

3. In an oven-proof skillet, Brown the chicken. Add wine and herbs. Cook until the sauce reduces by half. Then add 1 1/2 cups water and bring to a boil.

4. Cover and bake for 45 minutes. Stir in lemon juice before serving.

CALORIES	CARBS	SUGAR	FAT	PROTEIN	SODIUM
81	1.2	0.5	0.3	11.0	57
KCAL	GRAMS	GRAMS	GRAMS	GRAMS	MILLIGRAMS

INDONESIAN COCONUT CHICKEN OPOR

 SERVES 8

 PREP TIME 5 MINUTES

 COOK TIME 60 MINUTES

1. Blend all ingredients for the opor paste except lemongrass until smooth.

2. Brown the chicken. Then Brown the Tofu. Set aside.

3. Sauté the paste for 1 minute. Then add all ingredients except coconut milk. Add 4 cups of water. Bring to a boil then reduce to low. Cover and simmer for 45 minutes or until chicken is tender.

4. Stir in coconut milk and simmer, uncovered, for another 10 minutes.

Main Ingredients

- 1 pound chicken tender
- 10 ounce firm tofu, cut into bite-size pieces
- 1 1/2 cups light coconut milk
- 1/2 cups low sodium chicken broth
- Nonstick Cooking Spray

Opor Paste

- 10 shallots
- 10 cloves garlic
- 3 fresh bay leaves
- 2 lemongrass
- 1 tablespoon freshly grated ginger
- 2 teaspoons coriander powder
- 1 teaspoon ground turmeric
- 1/2 teaspoon salt
- 1/4 teaspoon pepper

CALORIES	CARBS	SUGAR	FAT	PROTEIN	SODIUM
136	9.0	1.1	4.1	15.5	226
KCAL	GRAMS	GRAMS	GRAMS	GRAMS	MILLIGRAMS

ITALIAN STUFFED CHICKEN BREAST

 SERVES
8

 PREP TIME
20
MINUTES

 COOK TIME
45
MINUTES

- **4** boneless, skinless chicken breasts, pounded
- **2** plum tomatoes, diced
- **2** red peppers, chopped
- **1 1/2 cups** marinara sauce
- **1 cup** fat-free shredded mozzarella cheese
- **2 tablespoons** chopped fresh basil
- **1 1/2 tablespoons** chopped fresh oregano
- salt and pepper to taste

1. Preheat the oven to 375°F.

2. Season the chicken with salt and pepper.

3. Cook tomatoes, peppers and herbs until hot. Remove from heat and stir in half the cheese. Season with salt and pepper.

4. Divide the mixture onto each chicken breast. Roll up and put in a baking dish.

5. Spread the marinara sauce on the chicken then top with the remaining cheese. Bake for 45 minutes.

CALORIES	CARBS	SUGAR	FAT	PROTEIN	SODIUM
104	5.5	1.7	1.0	16.9	327
KCAL	GRAMS	GRAMS	GRAMS	GRAMS	MILLIGRAMS

WHITE BEAN AND CHICKEN CHILI

 SERVES
8

 PREP TIME
40
MINUTES

 COOK TIME
25
MINUTES

1. Season the chicken with salt and pepper. Spray a large skillet. Brown the chicken. Set aside.

2. Sauté onion until fragrant. Add garlic, chili, cumin, coriander and chili powder. Cook for 1 minute. Add chicken and broth back to the pot. Cover and simmer for 30 minutes.

3. Remove the chicken and add the white beans. Shred the chicken and return to the pot. Simmer for 5-10 minutes until the sauce reduces to desired consistency.

- **1 pound** chicken tender
- 1 15.5-ounce **can** white beans, rinsed and drained
- **2 ounces** diced green chilies
- **1 cup** chopped onion
- 1 poblano chili, seeded and chopped
- **2 cloves** garlic, minced
- **2 cups** low sodium chicken broth
- **1 teaspoon** chili powder
- **1 teaspoon** ground cumin
- **1 teaspoon** ground coriander
- salt and pepper to taste

CALORIES	CARBS	SUGAR	FAT	PROTEIN	SODIUM
115	12.0	1.7	0.6	15.2	322
KCAL	GRAMS	GRAMS	GRAMS	GRAMS	MILLIGRAMS

NORTHERN ITALIAN CHICKEN STEW

SERVES
8

PREP TIME
10
MINUTES

COOK TIME
60
MINUTES

- **1 pound** chicken tender
- **1/2 cup** chopped onion
- **1/2 cup** sliced carrot
- **1/2 cup** sliced red bell pepper
- **1 cup** crushed tomatoes
- **2 cloves** garlic, minced
- **1** bay leave
- **2 tablespoons** dry white wine
- **1 tablespoon** chopped fresh parsley
- **1 teaspoon** minced rosemary

1. Season the chicken with salt and pepper. Spray a large skillet. Brown the chicken. Set aside.

2. Sauté the onion, carrot, bell peppers, garlic, bay leave and rosemary until fragrant. Add wine, tomato and chicken. Bring to a boil then reduce to low. Cover and simmer for 30 minutes.

CALORIES	CARBS	SUGAR	FAT	PROTEIN	SODIUM
77	4.8	2.4	0.3	11.9	145
KCAL	GRAMS	GRAMS	GRAMS	GRAMS	MILLIGRAMS

MUSTARD AND WINE BRAISED CHICKEN

SERVES **8**	**PREP TIME** **10** MINUTES	**COOK TIME** **60** MINUTES

1. Preheat the oven to 375°F.

2. Season the chicken with salt and pepper. Spray a large skillet. Brown the chicken. Set aside.

3. Sauté onion, garlic and shallots until fragrant. Add chicken, wine, mustard and broth back to the pot. Cover and bake for 45 minutes.

- **1 pound** chicken tender
- **2** shallots, chopped
- **2 cloves** garlic, minced
- **3/4 cup** low sodium chicken broth
- **1/2 cup** dry white wine
- **2 tablespoons** mustard
- **1 tablespoon** chopped fresh thyme
- salt and pepper to taste

CALORIES	CARBS	SUGAR	FAT	PROTEIN	SODIUM
71	1.6	0.6	0.3	11.4	105
KCAL	GRAMS	GRAMS	GRAMS	GRAMS	MILLIGRAMS

YAKITORI CHICKEN

 SERVES
8

 PREP TIME
8
HOURS

 COOK TIME
10
MINUTES

- **1 pound** chicken tender

- **2** green onions, chopped

- **1/2 cup** fat-free low sodium chicken broth

- **1/4 cup** sherry cooking wine

- **3 tablespoons** low sodium soy sauce

- **1 tablespoon** grated ginger

- **2 cloves** garlic, minced

1. In a large resealable bag, add all ingredients. Seal and shake the bag to mix well. Marinate overnight.

2. Preheat the broiler. Thread the meat onto 16 skewers.

3. Broil 3-4 minutes on each side.

CALORIES	CARBS	SUGAR	FAT	PROTEIN	SODIUM
64	1.1	0.2	0.3	11.6	343
KCAL	GRAMS	GRAMS	GRAMS	GRAMS	MILLIGRAMS

TUNA POKE

SERVES
4

PREP TIME
5
MINUTES

COOK TIME
5
MINUTES

1. In a medium bowl, combine all ingredients and serve.

- **1/2 pound** sushi grade tuna, cubed

- **1/4 cup** finely chopped green onion

- **2 tablespoons** low sodium soy sauce

- **1 teaspoon** lime juice

- **1 teaspoon** roasted sesame seed

CALORIES	CARBS	SUGAR	FAT	PROTEIN	SODIUM
91	1.0	0.0	2.4	14.7	310
KCAL	GRAMS	GRAMS	GRAMS	GRAMS	MILLIGRAMS

BROILED CURRY SALMON

 SERVES
4

 PREP TIME
10
MINUTES

 COOK TIME
10
MINUTES

- **2** salmon fillets (6-ounce each)

- **1 teaspoon** curry powder

- **1 teaspoon** garlic powder

- **1/2 teaspoon** cumin

- **1/4 teaspoon** salt

1. Preheat the broiler.

2. Mix the spice in a small bowl. Rub the spice evenly on the salmon.

3. Broil for 8-12 minutes.

CALORIES	CARBS	SUGAR	FAT	PROTEIN	SODIUM
80	0.9	0.0	0.9	18.2	256
KCAL	GRAMS	GRAMS	GRAMS	GRAMS	MILLIGRAMS

PORTOBELLO TUNA MELT

 SERVES 4

 PREP TIME 5 MINUTES

 COOK TIME 20 MINUTES

1. Preheat the broiler

2. In a medium bowl, combine tuna, mayonnaise, sour cream, onion and season with salt and pepper

3. Divide the tuna mixture on the mushroom.

4. Place a slice of tomato on each mushroom. Then Top with mozzarella cheese.

5. Place the mushroom on a rack and broil for 10-15 minutes until the cheese turns golden brown.

- 4 Portobello Mushroom, Gills and stems removed
- 1 5-ounce **can** tuna in water, drained
- **4 slices** tomatoes
- **1/4 cup** chopped onion
- **1/4 cup** low fat mayonnaise
- **1/4 cup** fat-free sour cream
- **1/4 cup** fat-free parmesan cheese
- **3/4 cup** fat-free mozzarella cheese
- salt and pepper to taste

CALORIES	CARBS	SUGAR	FAT	PROTEIN	SODIUM
137	14.8	3.7	1.8	17.5	620
KCAL	GRAMS	GRAMS	GRAMS	GRAMS	MILLIGRAMS

BUFFALO RANCH SALMON

SERVES
4

PREP TIME
10
MINUTES

COOK TIME
15
MINUTES

- **2** salmon fillets (6-ounce each)

- **2 tablespoon** whole wheat breadcrumbs

- **2 tablespoons** buffalo sauce

- **1 tablespoons** fat-free ranch seasoning

- **1/4 teaspoon** salt

- **1/4 teaspoon** pepper

1. Preheat the oven to 425°F.

2. In a small bowl, combine buffalo sauce, ranch seasoning, salt and pepper.

3. Spread the sauce on each salmon fillets. Sprinkle the breadcrumbs on top of each fillet.

4. Bake for 15 minutes.

CALORIES	CARBS	SUGAR	FAT	PROTEIN	SODIUM
95	2.6	0.4	1.6	18.4	469
KCAL	GRAMS	GRAMS	GRAMS	GRAMS	MILLIGRAMS

LEMON GLAZED SALMON

 SERVES
4

 PREP TIME
5
MINUTES

 COOK TIME
20
MINUTES

1. Brown the salmon fillet. Set aside.

2. Sauté garlic until fragrant.

3. Add lemon zest, lemon juice and broth. Simmer on low until reduces by half. Season with salt and pepper.

4. Return the Salmon. Simmer until the salmon is cooked through. Sprinkle parsley and serve.

- **2** salmon fillets (6-ounce each)

- **1** lemon, thinly sliced

- **2 tablespoons** lemon juice

- **1 tablespoon** lemon zest

- **3 cloves** garlic, minced

- **1 cup** fat-free low sodium chicken broth

- **2 tablespoons** chopped fresh parsley

- salt and pepper to taste

- Non-stick Cooking Spray

CALORIES	CARBS	SUGAR	FAT	PROTEIN	SODIUM
83	1.8	0.2	0.8	18.7	132
KCAL	GRAMS	GRAMS	GRAMS	GRAMS	MILLIGRAMS

SMOKED SALMON SCRAMBLE

 SERVES
8

 PREP TIME
10
MINUTES

 COOK TIME
15
MINUTES

- **4 ounces** smoked salmon

- **2** large eggs and **4** egg whites

- **2 cups** baby spinach

- **2 cloves** garlic, minced

- **2 tablespoons** low fat cheddar cheese

- salt and pepper to taste

- Nonstick Cooking Spray

1. Sauté garlic and spinach until fragrant.

2. In a medium bowl, whisk the eggs and cheese. Season with salt and pepper.

3. Add the egg mixture. Scramble for 30 seconds.

4. Add salmon. Scramble for until eggs are cooked through.

CALORIES	CARBS	SUGAR	FAT	PROTEIN	SODIUM
97	1.4	0.4	3.9	13.1	320
KCAL	GRAMS	GRAMS	GRAMS	GRAMS	MILLIGRAMS

TILAPIA TOMATO ALFREDO

 SERVES
8

 PREP TIME
5
MINUTES

 COOK TIME
20
MINUTES

1. Season the fish with salt and pepper. Set aside.

2. Sauté garlic and onion until fragrant.

3. Add soup, milk and tomatoes. Cook until bubbly. Add Fish and bring it to a boil. Then reduce to low and simmer for 10-15 minutes.

- **1 pound** tilapia fillet, cut into 2-inch pieces

- 1 10.5-ounce **can** fat-free condensed cream of mushroom soup

- 1 10-ounce **can** diced tomatoes, drained

- **1/2 cup** chopped onion

- **3 cloves** garlic, minced

- **1/2 cup** skim milk

- **2 tablespoons** chopped fresh parsley

- salt and pepper to taste

- Nonstick Cooking Spray

CALORIES	CARBS	SUGAR	FAT	PROTEIN	SODIUM
84	5.8	1.8	2.1	11.3	324
KCAL	GRAMS	GRAMS	GRAMS	GRAMS	MILLIGRAMS

SPICY HALIBUT PARMESAN

 SERVES
8

 PREP TIME
15
MINUTES

 COOK TIME
10
MINUTES

- **1 pound** skinless halibut fillets

- **1** green onion, chopped

- **1/2 cup** fat-free parmesan cheese

- **1 1/2 tablespoons** fat-free mayonnaise

- **1 tablespoons** lemon juice

- **1 teaspoon** hot sauce

- **1/4 teaspoon** salt

- Nonstick Cooking Spray

1. Preheat the oven to 425°F.

2. In a medium bowl, combine all ingredients except fish.

3. Season the fish with salt and pepper. Place the fish on a baking dish. Bake for 10 minutes.

4. Spread the cheese mixture on top and bake for another 5 minutes or until cheese are bubbly and golden brown.

CALORIES	CARBS	SUGAR	FAT	PROTEIN	SODIUM
68	3.8	0.3	0.5	12.5	270
KCAL	GRAMS	GRAMS	GRAMS	GRAMS	MILLIGRAMS

ASIAN SALMON MEATBALLS

 SERVES
6

 PREP TIME
5
MINUTES

 COOK TIME
25
MINUTES

1. Preheat the oven to 350°F.

2. In a large bowl, combine all ingredients. Divide the mixture into 12 meatballs. Apply nonstick cooking spray.

3. Bake for 15-18 minutes.

- **12 ounces** canned pink salmon, drained

- **1/2 cup** whole wheat breadcrumbs

- **2** green onions, finely chopped

- **2 cloves** garlic, minced

- **1/2 tablespoon** grated ginger

- **1** egg

- **1/4 teaspoon** salt

- **1/4 teaspoon** ground black pepper

CALORIES	CARBS	SUGAR	FAT	PROTEIN	SODIUM
99	5.6	0.5	2.5	14.2	296
KCAL	GRAMS	GRAMS	GRAMS	GRAMS	MILLIGRAMS

SPICY PEANUT SALMON BURGER

SERVES **6**	**PREP TIME** **5** MINUTES	**COOK TIME** **25** MINUTES

- **12 ounces** canned pink salmon, drained

- **1/2 cup** whole wheat breadcrumbs

- **2** green onions, finely chopped

- **1 1/2 tablespoons** low sodium soy sauce

- **2 tablespoons** powdered peanut butter

- **1 tablespoon** hot sauce

- **1/4 cup** fat-free Greek yogurt

1. Preheat the oven to 350°F.

2. In a large bowl, combine all ingredients. Divide the mixture into 12 patties. Apply nonstick cooking spray.

3. Bake for 15-18 minutes.

CALORIES	CARBS	SUGAR	FAT	PROTEIN	SODIUM
120 KCAL	**7.0** GRAMS	**0.9** GRAMS	**3.4** GRAMS	**16.1** GRAMS	**477** MILLIGRAMS

ASIAN GINGER CATFISH

	SERVES		PREP TIME		COOK TIME
	8		**15** MINUTES		**20** MINUTES

1. Sauté ginger until golden brown. Sear the fish. 3 minutes on each side. Set aside.

2. Sauté garlic, green onion, onion and bell peppers until fragrant. Add fish sauce, soy sauce and oyster sauce. Return the fish and bury the fish in the sauce and cook for 3-5 more minutes.

- **1 pound** catfish fillet, cut into 2-inch pieces
- **4 ounces** fresh ginger, peeled and cut into thin strips
- **1/2 cup** chopped onion
- **1/2 cup** sliced red bell peppers
- **2** green onions, chopped
- **2 tablespoons** fish sauce
- **1 tablespoons** oyster sauce
- **1 tablespoon** low-sodium soy sauce
- Nonstick Cooking Spray

CALORIES	CARBS	SUGAR	FAT	PROTEIN	SODIUM
123 KCAL	**3.5** GRAMS	**1.2** GRAMS	**1.0** GRAMS	**12.3** GRAMS	**518** MILLIGRAMS

CHEESY TUNA CASSEROLE

 SERVES
8

 PREP TIME
10
MINUTES

 COOK TIME
30
MINUTES

- 3 5-ounce **cans** tuna in water, drained
- **1** medium head cauliflower, cut into florets
- **1 cup** diced onion
- **1 cup** low-fat alfredo sauce
- **1 cup** skim milk
- **1/2 cup** fat-free parmesan cheese
- **1 cup** fat-free mozzarella cheese
- Nonstick Cooking Spray

1. Preheat the broiler

2. In a large pot, add enough water to cover the cauliflower. Cook until cauliflower is soft. Drain and mash the cauliflower. Season with salt and pepper.

3. Sauté onion until fragrant. Add milk and alfredo sauce. Stir in the parmesan cheese, tuna and cauliflower mash. Adjust seasoning if needed.

4. Top with mozzarella cheese and broil until the cheese is golden brown and bubbly.

CALORIES	CARBS	SUGAR	FAT	PROTEIN	SODIUM
148	12.0	4.2	3.5	18.0	670
KCAL	GRAMS	GRAMS	GRAMS	GRAMS	MILLIGRAMS

MEDITERRANEAN WHITE FISH

 SERVES
8

 PREP TIME
15
MINUTES

 COOK TIME
30
MINUTES

1. Preheat the oven to 425°F.

2. Season the fish with salt and pepper. Place the fish on a baking dish. Set aside.

3. Sauté garlic and onion until fragrant. Then add tomatoes and cook until tender. Add capers, olives, wine, oregano and basil. Reduce to low heat. Stir in cheese. Cook on low until the sauce reduces by half.

4. Spread the sauce on the fish. Bake for 10-15 minutes.

- **1 pound** white fish fillet
- **5** plum tomatoes, diced
- **1/2 cup** chopped onion
- **2 cloves** garlic, minced
- **4 tablespoons** capers
- **6** black olives, pitted and chopped
- **1/4 cup** dry white wine
- **3 tablespoons** fat-free parmesan cheese
- **1/2 teaspoon** dried basil
- pinch of dried oregano

CALORIES	CARBS	SUGAR	FAT	PROTEIN	SODIUM
98	3.8	1.8	1.3	14.8	340
KCAL	GRAMS	GRAMS	GRAMS	GRAMS	MILLIGRAMS

GARLIC HERB TUNA STEAK

 SERVES
4

 PREP TIME
40
MINUTES

 COOK TIME
10
MINUTES

- **2** tuna steak (6-ounce each)

- **2 cloves** garlic, minced

- **2 tablespoons** lemon juice

- **2 teaspoons** minced fresh thyme

- **1/4 teaspoon** salt

- **1/4 teaspoon** pepper

1. In a large resealable plastic bag, combine all ingredients. Put in the refrigerator and marinade for 30 minutes.

2. Preheat the broiler.

3. Discard the marinade, broil the tuna steak 3-4 minutes on each side.

CALORIES	CARBS	SUGAR	FAT	PROTEIN	SODIUM
95	1.3	0.2	0.8	19.7	173
KCAL	GRAMS	GRAMS	GRAMS	GRAMS	MILLIGRAMS

SPICY HUMMUS TUNA CAKE

SERVES
12

PREP TIME
20
MINUTES

COOK TIME
40
MINUTES

1. Preheat the oven to 350°F.

2. In a large bowl, combine all ingredients.

3. Spray a muffin tin. Divide the mixture into 12 cups.

4. Bake for 40 minutes.

- **3** 5-ounce **cans** tuna in water, drained

- **1 cup** roasted red pepper hummus

- **2 cloves** garlic, minced

- **1** green onion, chopped

- **1** jalapeno pepper, seeded and chopped

- **2** large eggs

- **1/4 teaspoon** salt

CALORIES	CARBS	SUGAR	FAT	PROTEIN	SODIUM
85	4.3	0.1	3.8	8.7	312
KCAL	GRAMS	GRAMS	GRAMS	GRAMS	MILLIGRAMS

BALSAMIC PORK TENDERLOIN

 SERVES **6**

 PREP TIME **15** MINUTES

 COOK TIME **10** MINUTES

- **1 pound** pork tenderloin, cut into 1.5-inch piece

- **1/4 cup** fat-free low sodium chicken broth

- **2 tablespoons** balsamic vinegar

- **2 tablespoons** whole wheat flour

- **1 teaspoon** capers

- **1 teaspoon** lemon zest

- **1/2 teaspoon** salt

- **1/4 teaspoon** pepper

1. In a small bowl, mix together flour, salt and pepper. Coat the pork in the mixture. Shake off excess flour.

2. Brown the pork. Add vinegar and broth. Bring to a boil and reduce to low. Simmer for 4-5 minutes until pork is cooked through.

3. Remove the pork. Add lemon zest and capers. Simmer until the desired consistency. Pour the sauce over the pork and serve.

CALORIES	CARBS	SUGAR	FAT	PROTEIN	SODIUM
77	2.7	0.8	1.4	15.0	550
KCAL	GRAMS	GRAMS	GRAMS	GRAMS	MILLIGRAMS

PORK AND BROCCOLI STIR FRY

 SERVES
8

 PREP TIME
5
MINUTES

 COOK TIME
20
MINUTES

1. In a large bowl, mix the pork with soy sauce, garlic, ground ginger and crushed red pepper. Set aside to marinate.

2. Blanch the broccoli in a pot of boiling water until slightly softened. Drain and set aside.

3. Sauté onion until fragrant. Set aside.

4. Add the pork without the marinate. Cook until cook through.

5. Dissolve the flour in the broth. Add broth and sauce. Cook until sauce thickens.

6. Add the broccoli and onion. Stir fry for 2-3 minutes until cooked through.

- **1 pound** pork tenderloin, thinly sliced
- **12 ounces** broccoli floret
- **1 cup** sliced onion
- **2 cloves** garlic, minced
- **1 cup** fat free low sodium chicken broth
- **2 tablespoons** low sodium soy sauce
- **1 tablespoon** whole wheat flour
- **1/4 teaspoon** ground ginger
- **1/8 teaspoon** crushed red pepper
- Nonstick Cooking Spray

CALORIES	CARBS	SUGAR	FAT	PROTEIN	SODIUM
78	6.0	1.3	1.2	13.0	364
KCAL	GRAMS	GRAMS	GRAMS	GRAMS	MILLIGRAMS

PORK CHOPS IN MUSHROOM SAUCE

 SERVES **8**

 PREP TIME **10** MINUTES

 COOK TIME **40** MINUTES

- **4** pork chops (4-ounce each)

- **1** 10.5-ounce **can** fat-free condensed cream of mushroom soup

- **2 cups** sliced mushrooms

- **1 cup** chopped onion

- **2 cloves** garlic, minced

- **2 tablespoons** dry white wine

- pinch of thyme

- salt and pepper to taste

- Nonstick Cooking Spray

1. Season the pork chops with salt and pepper.

2. Sauté garlic and onion until fragrant. Set aside.

3. Brown the pork chops. Add all ingredients and mix well. Cover and simmer on low for 20-25 minutes

CALORIES	CARBS	SUGAR	FAT	PROTEIN	SODIUM
107	6.0	0.9	3.1	13.1	521
KCAL	GRAMS	GRAMS	GRAMS	GRAMS	MILLIGRAMS

PORK CHOPS IN CREAMY ONION SAUCE

 SERVES
8

 PREP TIME
10
MINUTES

 COOK TIME
40
MINUTES

1. Season the pork chops with salt and pepper.

2. Sauté garlic and onion until fragrant. Set aside.

3. Brown the pork chops. Add broth. Cover and simmer on low for 20-25 minutes.

4. Remove the pork chops. Simmer the sauce until reduces by half. Stir in sour cream and paprika. Pour the sauce over the pork chops and serve.

- **4 pork chops** (4-ounce each)
- **1 1/2 cups** chopped onion
- **1/2 cup** fat-free low sodium chicken broth
- **1 clove** garlic, minced
- **3/4 cup** fat-free sour cream
- **2 teaspoons** paprika
- salt and pepper to taste
- Nonstick Cooking Spray

CALORIES	CARBS	SUGAR	FAT	PROTEIN	SODIUM
95	5.5	2.8	2.4	13.6	153
KCAL	GRAMS	GRAMS	GRAMS	GRAMS	MILLIGRAMS

PORK STROGANOFF

 SERVES
8

 PREP TIME
10
MINUTES

 COOK TIME
40
MINUTES

- **1 pound** pork tenderloin, cut into thin strips
- **2 cups** sliced mushrooms
- **1 cup** chopped onion
- **2 cloves** garlic, minced
- **1/2 cup** fat-free low-sodium chicken broth
- **1 cup** fat-free half and half
- **2 tablespoons** fat free sour cream
- **1 tablespoon** mustard
- **1 teaspoon** paprika
- **1 teaspoon** tomato paste
- **1 teaspoon** chili powder
- **1 teaspoon** lemon juice
- salt and pepper to taste

1. Season the pork chops with salt and pepper.

2. Sauté garlic, onion and mushrooms until fragrant. Set aside.

3. Brown the pork chops. Add broth. Cover and simmer on low for 20-25 minutes.

4. Remove the pork chops.

5. Stir in cream, mustard, tomato paste, lemon juice and other seasoning. Pour the sauce over the pork

CALORIES	CARBS	SUGAR	FAT	PROTEIN	SODIUM
93	7.3	2.7	1.5	13.6	448
KCAL	GRAMS	GRAMS	GRAMS	GRAMS	MILLIGRAMS

VINEGAR MUSTARD GLAZED HAM LOAF

 SERVES
16

 PREP TIME
10
MINUTES

 COOK TIME
90
MINUTES

1. Preheat the oven to 350°F.

2. In a large bowl, combine ham, pork, eggs, evaporated milk, salt and pepper. Spray a 9x13 baking dish. Place the mixture in the dish. Bake for 90 minutes.

3. In a small bowl, mix together vinegar, mustard and truvia. Pour the mixture on top of the loaf in the last 15 minutes.

- **2 pounds** extra lean ham
- **1 pound** extra lean ground pork
- **2** eggs
- **1 cup** whole wheat breadcrumbs
- **1 cup** low-fat evaporated milk
- **1/3 cup** Truvia brown sugar
- **1/4 cup** apple cider vinegar
- **1 tablespoon** mustard powder
- **1/4 teaspoon** salt
- **1/4 teaspoon** ground black pepper

CALORIES	CARBS	SUGAR	FAT	PROTEIN	SODIUM
146	9.6	4.3	4.7	17.3	755
KCAL	GRAMS	GRAMS	GRAMS	GRAMS	MILLIGRAMS

GARLIC LEMON SCALLOPS

 SERVES
8

 PREP TIME
5
MINUTES

 COOK TIME
10
MINUTES

- **1 pound** sea scallops, patted dry

- **6 cloves** garlic, minced

- **2 scallions**, finely chopped

- **1 lemon**, juice only

- **1 tablespoon** whole wheat flour

- **1/4 teaspoon** salt

- pinch of ground sage

- Nonstick cooking spray

1. In a bowl, mix scallops with flour and salt.

2. Spray a large skillet, Sear the scallops until golden brown. Set aside.

3. sauté garlic and scallion until fragrant. Add lemon juice and return scallops. Stir well and cook for 30 seconds. Sprinkle with parsley and serve.

CALORIES	CARBS	SUGAR	FAT	PROTEIN	SODIUM
72	5.2	0.2	0.5	11.7	450
KCAL	GRAMS	GRAMS	GRAMS	GRAMS	MILLIGRAMS

SCALLOPS IN JALAPENO WHISKY CREAM SAUCE

 SERVES 8

 PREP TIME 5 MINUTES

 COOK TIME 10 MINUTES

1. In a bowl, mix scallops with flour and 1/4 teaspoon salt. Spray a large skillet, Sear the scallops until golden brown. Set aside.

2. sauté garlic and pepper until fragrant. Add whisky and cook for 1 minute. Stir in cream and bring to a simmer. Season with salt and pepper.

3. Pour sauce over scallops. Sprinkle with chopped cilantro and serve.

- **1 pound** sea scallops, patted dry
- **2 cloves** garlic, minced
- **2** jalapeno pepper, seeded and finely chopped
- **1 cup** fat-free half and half
- **1/2 cup** chopped fresh cilantro
- **1/8 cup** bourbon whiskey
- **1 tablespoon** whole wheat flour
- **3/4 teaspoon** salt
- **1/2 teaspoon** ground black pepper

CALORIES	CARBS	SUGAR	FAT	PROTEIN	SODIUM
96	7.1	1.7	0.9	12.4	623
KCAL	GRAMS	GRAMS	GRAMS	GRAMS	MILLIGRAMS

LOWCOUNTRY SHRIMPS

 SERVES
8

 PREP TIME
5
MINUTES

 COOK TIME
15
MINUTES

- **1 pound** fresh shrimps, peeled and deveined

- 1 6.5-ounce **link** lean turkey sausage, sliced

- **1 cup** sliced bell pepper

- **2 cloves** garlic, minced

- **1 teaspoon** old bay seasoning

- **1/4 teaspoon** ground black pepper

- **1/4 cup** water

- Nonstick Cooking Spray

1. In a large bowl, season shrimp with old bay seasoning and black pepper. Set aside.

2. Spray a large skillet, sauté garlic until fragrant. Add sausage and cook until crispy. Add shrimp and water. Cook while stirring until cook through.

CALORIES	CARBS	SUGAR	FAT	PROTEIN	SODIUM
75	1.2	0.4	1.6	13.5	448
KCAL	GRAMS	GRAMS	GRAMS	GRAMS	MILLIGRAMS

CHEESY ONION SCALLOPS

 SERVES
8

 PREP TIME
5
MINUTES

 COOK TIME
15
MINUTES

1. Preheat the broiler.

2. In a bowl, mix scallops with flour and 1/4 teaspoon salt. Spray an oven-proof skillet. Sear the scallops until golden brown. Set aside.

3. sauté garlic, onion and shallots until fragrant. Add wine and water. Simmer until the sauce reduces by half. Season with salt and pepper.

4. Stir in the scallops. Top with cheese and broil for 3-5 minutes until cheese turns golden brown.

- **1 pound** sea scallops, patted dry
- **2 cloves** garlic, minced
- **2** shallots, chopped
- **1/4 cup** chopped onion
- **3/4 cup** white wine
- **1/4 cup** water
- **1/4 cup** fat-free parmesan cheese
- **1** bay leave
- **2 tablespoons** chopped fresh thyme
- **1 tablespoon** whole wheat flour
- salt and pepper to taste

CALORIES	CARBS	SUGAR	FAT	PROTEIN	SODIUM
94	6.0	0.3	0.5	12.1	460
KCAL	GRAMS	GRAMS	GRAMS	GRAMS	MILLIGRAMS

SHRIMP À LA GRECQUE

 SERVES
8

 PREP TIME
5
MINUTES

 COOK TIME
20
MINUTES

- **1 pound** fresh shrimps, peeled and deveined

- **1 1/2 cups** canned crushed tomatoes, drained

- **3 ounces** fat-free feta cheese, cubed

- **2 cloves** garlic, minced

- **1/2 cup** dry white wine

- **2 tablespoons** chopped fresh parsley

- **1/2 teaspoon** dried oregano, crushed

- **1/4 teaspoon** salt

- **1/4 teaspoon** ground black pepper

1. Spray a large skillet, sauté garlic until fragrant. Add tomatoes, wine, oregano, salt and pepper. Cook until sauce thickens.

2. Add shrimp, cook while stirring until cook through. Remove from heat. Add cheese and parsley before serving.

CALORIES	CARBS	SUGAR	FAT	PROTEIN	SODIUM
97	4.3	1.7	0.9	14.1	507
KCAL	GRAMS	GRAMS	GRAMS	GRAMS	MILLIGRAMS

CRAB IMPERIAL

SERVES
8

PREP TIME
10
MINUTES

COOK TIME
20
MINUTES

1. Preheat the oven to 400°F.

2. In a large bowl, combine all

3. ingredients except paprika and cilantro.

4. Transfer the mixture to a baking dish. Sprinkle Paprika and bake for 20 minutes. Garnish with fresh cilantro and serve.

- **1 pound** crab meat
- **1/2 cup** chopped bell peppers
- **1/2 cup** chopped celery
- **2** egg whites, beaten
- **1/2** lemon, juice only
- **1 cup** fat-free plain yogurt
- **2 tablespoons** chopped fresh cilantro
- **1 teaspoon** dry mustard
- **1/4 teaspoon** salt
- **1/4 teaspoon** Worcestershire sauce
- **1/8 teaspoon** chili powder
- **1/8 teaspoon** paprika

CALORIES	CARBS	SUGAR	FAT	PROTEIN	SODIUM
76	**10.8**	**4.9**	**0.6**	**7.4**	**423**
KCAL	GRAMS	GRAMS	GRAMS	GRAMS	MILLIGRAMS

STEAMED CLAMS IN GARLIC WINE SAUCE

 SERVES **5**

 PREP TIME **10** MINUTES

 COOK TIME **25** MINUTES

- **50** small clams, scrubbed
- **1 cup** white wine
- **8 cloves** garlic, minced
- **1/2 cup** chopped fresh parsley
- **1 tablespoon** butter
- salt and pepper to taste
- Nonstick Cooking Spray

1. Spray a large skillet, sauté garlic until fragrant. Add wine. Simmer until sauce reduces by half, about 15 minutes.

2. Add clams, cover and steam until clams begin to open, about 5 minutes.

3. Stir in butter and cover. Steam until most clams open, about 5 minutes. Season with salt and pepper. Sprinkle with parsley and serve.

CALORIES	CARBS	SUGAR	FAT	PROTEIN	SODIUM
168	5.7	0.1	3.6	18.9	111
KCAL	GRAMS	GRAMS	GRAMS	GRAMS	MILLIGRAMS

MUSSELS IN MARINARA SAUCE

 SERVES
6

 PREP TIME
10
MINUTES

 COOK TIME
30
MINUTES

1. Spray a large skillet, sauté garlic until fragrant. Add wine. Simmer until sauce reduces by half, about 15 minutes.

2. Add tomatoes and green onion and cook for 4-5 minutes until softens.

3. Add mussels. Cover and cook until mussels start to open, about 5 minutes. Stir in butter. cover and cook until most mussels open.

4. Sprinkle with parsley and serve.

- **50** mussels, scrubbed and debearded

- **6 cloves** garlic, minced

- **3** plum tomatoes, chopped

- **3** green onion, chopped

- **1/2 cup** chopped fresh parsley

- **1 cup** white wine

- **1 tablespoon** butter

- salt and pepper to taste

- Nonstick Cooking Spray

CALORIES	CARBS	SUGAR	FAT	PROTEIN	SODIUM
174	8.1	1.3	4.9	16.9	410
KCAL	GRAMS	GRAMS	GRAMS	GRAMS	MILLIGRAMS

CREAMY CAJUN SHRIMPS

SERVES
12

PREP TIME
10
MINUTES

COOK TIME
30
MINUTES

- **1 1/2 pounds** fresh shrimps, peeled and deveined

- **1/2 cup** sliced mushrooms

- **2** green onions, chopped

- **1/4 cup** low-fat alfredo sauce

- **1/4 cup** chopped fresh parsley

- **1/4 cup** skim milk

- **1/4 cup** fat-free grated parmesan cheese

- **1 tablespoon** Cajun seasoning

- salt and pepper to taste

- Nonstick Cooking Spray

1. Preheat the oven to 350°F.

2. Season the shrimp with Cajun seasoning, salt and pepper.

3. Spray a large skillet, sauté mushrooms and green onion until fragrant. Add shrimp and sauté until cooked through. Transfer to a baking Dish.

4. Add alfredo sauce and skim milk to the pan and stir to combine.

Pour the sauce over the shrimps. Sprinkle with parmesan cheese and bake for 20 minutes.

CALORIES	CARBS	SUGAR	FAT	PROTEIN	SODIUM
69	1.2	0.4	1.3	12.7	485
KCAL	GRAMS	GRAMS	GRAMS	GRAMS	MILLIGRAMS

MARYLAND CRAB CAKE

SERVES
8

PREP TIME
60
MINUTES

COOK TIME
15
MINUTES

1. In a large bowl, combine crabmeat, egg, half of the breadcrumbs, mayonnaise, mustard, Worcestershire sauce and all seasoning. Refrigerate for 1 hour.

2. Spread the remaining breadcrumbs on a large plate.

3. Divide the crab mixture into 8 portions and shape into patties. Coat with bread crumbs on each side.

4. Spray a pan, cook the crab cakes until golden brown on each side.

- **1 pound** crab meat
- **1/2 cup** whole wheat breadcrumbs, divided
- **2 tablespoons** fat-free mayonnaise
- **1 egg**, beaten
- **1/2 teaspoon** Dijon Mustard
- **1/2 teaspoon** Old Bay seasoning
- **1/4 teaspoon** Worcestershire sauce
- **1/4 teaspoon** salt
- **1/8 teaspoon** ground black pepper
- Nonstick cooking spray

CALORIES	CARBS	SUGAR	FAT	PROTEIN	SODIUM
69	4.1	0.6	0.7	11.5	346
KCAL	GRAMS	GRAMS	GRAMS	GRAMS	MILLIGRAMS

GRILLED TOMATO BASIL SHRIMPS

 SERVES
8

 PREP TIME
2
HOURS

 COOK TIME
15
MINUTES

- **1 pound** fresh shrimps, peeled and deveined

- **4 cloves** garlic, minced

- **3 tablespoons** tomato sauce

- **2 tablespoons** chopped fresh basil

- **1 tablespoons** red wine vinegar

- **1 tablespoon** olive oil

- **1/4 teaspoon** salt

- **1/8 teaspoon** cayenne pepper

- Nonstick Cooking Spray

1. In a large resealable bag, add all ingredients and mix well. Seal the bag and refrigerate for 2 hours to marinate.

2. Prepare the grill. Thread the shrimp onto skewers. Spray the Grill. Cook shrimp for 2-3 minutes on each side or until opaque

CALORIES	CARBS	SUGAR	FAT	PROTEIN	SODIUM
77	0.9	0.5	2.6	12.2	361
KCAL	GRAMS	GRAMS	GRAMS	GRAMS	MILLIGRAMS

GRILLED LEMON GINGER SHRIMPS

SERVES
8

PREP TIME
10
MINUTES

COOK TIME
50
MINUTES

1. In a large resealable bag, add all ingredients and mix well. Seal the bag and refrigerate for 2 hours to marinate.

2. Prepare the grill. Thread the shrimp onto skewers. Spray the Grill. Cook shrimp for 2-3 minutes on each side or until opaque

- **1 pound** fresh shrimps, peeled and deveined

- **4 cloves** garlic, minced

- **1/4 cup** lemon juice

- **1/4 cup** chopped fresh cilantro

- **3 tablespoons** grated ginger

- **1 teaspoon** paprika

- **1/4 teaspoon** salt

- **1/4 teaspoon** ground black pepper

CALORIES	CARBS	SUGAR	FAT	PROTEIN	SODIUM
66	1.9	0.3	1.0	12.4	345
KCAL	GRAMS	GRAMS	GRAMS	GRAMS	MILLIGRAMS

TACO SALAD

 SERVES
8

 PREP TIME
15
MINUTES

 COOK TIME
10
MINUTES

- **1 pound** 97/3 lean ground beef

- **1 head** romaine lettuce, chopped

- **2** medium tomatoes, chopped

- **8** green onions, green and white separated and chopped

- **1 1/2 cups** fat-free shredded cheddar cheese

- **1/2 cup** fat-free Greek Yogurt

- **1/2 cup** salsa

- **1 tablespoon** chili powder

- salt and pepper to taste

1. Brown the beef with white part of onions. Season with chili powder, salt and pepper.

2. In a large bowl, toss all ingredients except yogurt and salsa together. Spoon yogurt and salsa on the side and serve.

CALORIES	CARBS	SUGAR	FAT	PROTEIN	SODIUM
134	7.6	2.7	2.4	21.8	376
KCAL	GRAMS	GRAMS	GRAMS	GRAMS	MILLIGRAMS

ASIAN LETTUCE WRAP

 SERVES **8**

 PREP TIME **15** MINUTES

 COOK TIME **20** MINUTES

1. Spray a large skillet, sauté garlic, onion, green onion and water chestnut until fragrant. Drain the liquid and set aside.

2. Brown the beef. Then add all ingredients except lettuce. Stir well. Cook for another 2-3 minutes.

3. Divide the beef onto the lettuce leaves. Roll up and serve.

- **1 pound** 97/3 lean ground beef
- **1** 8-ounce **can** water chestnut, finely chopped
- **8** large romaine lettuce leaves
- **2 cloves** garlic, minced
- **1/2 cup** chopped onion
- **1/4 cup** chopped green onion
- **1/4 cup** hoisin sauce
- **2 tablespoons** low sodium soy sauce
- **2 tablespoon** rice wine vinegar
- **1 tablespoon** chili paste
- **1 tablespoon** grated ginger
- **1 tablespoon** sesame oil
- Nonstick cooking spray

CALORIES	CARBS	SUGAR	FAT	PROTEIN	SODIUM
121	9.0	3.5	4.1	13.0	351
KCAL	GRAMS	GRAMS	GRAMS	GRAMS	MILLIGRAMS

SHRIMP SALAD STUFFED TOMATOES

 SERVES
8

PREP TIME
35
MINUTES

 COOK TIME
/
MINUTES

- **1 pound** shrimp, peeled, deveined, cooked and chopped

- **4** large ripe tomatoes, cored

- **1 stalk** celery, chopped

- **1** shallot, minced

- **1/4 cup** chopped fresh basil

- **2 tablespoons** low-fat mayonnaise

- **1 tablespoon** white wine vinegar

- salt and pepper to taste

- pinch of paprika

1. In a medium bowl, combine shrimp, celery, shallots, basil, mayonnaise and vinegar. Season with salt and pepper.

2. Spoon the mixture into the tomatoes. Garnish with pinch of paprika and serve.

CALORIES	CARBS	SUGAR	FAT	PROTEIN	SODIUM
80	4.5	2.8	1.3	12.9	309
KCAL	GRAMS	GRAMS	GRAMS	GRAMS	MILLIGRAMS

SLOPPY JOE LETTUCE WRAP

SERVES
8

PREP TIME
10
MINUTES

COOK TIME
40
MINUTES

1. Spray a large skillet, sauté garlic, onion and bell pepper until fragrant. Drain the liquid and set aside.

2. Brown the beef. Then add all ingredients except lettuce. Stir well. Reduce to low heat and simmer for 25 minutes.

3. Divide the beef onto the lettuce leaves. Roll up and serve.

- **1 pound** 97/3 lean ground beef

- **8** large romaine lettuce leaves

- **3/4 cup** tomato sauce

- **1/4 cup** chopped onion

- **1/4 cup** chopped green bell peppers

- **2 cloves** garlic, minced.

- **1 teaspoon** yellow mustard

- **1 teaspoon** stevia

- salt and pepper to taste

- Nonstick Cooking Spray

CALORIES	CARBS	SUGAR	FAT	PROTEIN	SODIUM
82	3.6	1.6	2.2	12.8	155
KCAL	GRAMS	GRAMS	GRAMS	GRAMS	MILLIGRAMS

GARDEN SALAD WITH LEMON CHICKEN AND FETA

 SERVES
6

 PREP TIME
40
MINUTES

 COOK TIME
20
MINUTES

For Chicken:

- 2 boneless skinless chicken breasts
- 1/4 cup lemon juice
- 2 cloves garlic, minced
- 2 tablespoons chopped fresh dill
- 1/2 teaspoon salt
- 1/4 teaspoon ground black pepper
- Nonstick cooking spray

For salad:

- 1/2 medium seedless cucumber, chopped
- 2 medium tomatoes, chopped
- 3 ounces fat-free feta cheese, cubed
- 2 tablespoons lemon juice
- 1 tablespoon olive oil
- 1/2 teaspoon Dijon mustard
- 1/2 teaspoon stevia
- salt and pepper to taste

1. In a medium resealable bag, add all ingredients for the chicken. Seal and press to coat the marinade evenly. Refrigerate for 30 minutes. Discard the marinade and dry the chicken.

2. Sear the chicken until golden brown on one side. Flip, reduce to low heat, cover and cook for 10-15 minutes until cooked through. Set aside to cool. Then slice into bite size.

3. Combine lemon juice, olive oil, mustard and stevia. In a large bowl, toss all ingredients together and serve.

CALORIES	CARBS	SUGAR	FAT	PROTEIN	SODIUM
111	8.5	3.1	2.9	12.9	475
KCAL	GRAMS	GRAMS	GRAMS	GRAMS	MILLIGRAMS

BUFFALO CHICKEN LETTUCE WRAP

 SERVES
8

 PREP TIME
10
MINUTES

 COOK TIME
60
MINUTES

1. Brown the chicken tender on both sides.

2. Add broth and beer. Cover and simmer for 1 hour.

3. Shredd the chicken. Add the chicken and buffalo sauce to a pan. Cook for 2-3 minutes. Season with salt.

4. Divide the chicken onto lettuce leaves. Top with cheese. Roll up and serve

- **1 pound** chicken tender

- 8 large romaine lettuce leave

- **1 cup** fat free low-sodium chicken broth

- **3/4 cup** beer

- **3 tablespoons** buffalo wing sauce

- **1/2 cup** low-fat crumbled blue cheese

- salt and pepper to taste

CALORIES	CARBS	SUGAR	FAT	PROTEIN	SODIUM
92	2.0	1.0	2.1	13.1	285
KCAL	GRAMS	GRAMS	GRAMS	GRAMS	MILLIGRAMS

SEARED TANDOORI TOFU

 SERVES 5

 PREP TIME 5 MINUTES

 COOK TIME 10 MINUTES

- 1 14-ounce **block** extra firm tofu, sliced into 1/2-inch slices

- **1 tablespoon** cayenne pepper

- **1 tablespoon** cumin

- **1 tablespoon** turmeric

- **1 tablespoon** smoked paprika

- **1/2 teaspoon** salt

- **1/2 teaspoon** black pepper

- Nonstick Cooking Spray

1. In a small bowl, mix all spices and seasoning together.

2. Spray a skillet. Heat on medium. Coat one side of the tofu and place the tofu face down. Sear both side until golden brown, around 2-3 minutes each side.

CALORIES	CARBS	SUGAR	FAT	PROTEIN	SODIUM
95	3.2	0.1	4.2	7.8	239
KCAL	GRAMS	GRAMS	GRAMS	GRAMS	MILLIGRAMS

ITALIAN PORTOBELLO BAKE

 SERVES
12

 PREP TIME
15
MINUTES

 COOK TIME
15
MINUTES

1. Preheat the oven to 400°F.

2. Spray a large skillet, sauté mushrooms until fragrant. Season with salt and pepper. Transfer to a baking dish.

3. In a medium bowl, Mix tomatoes with all herbs. Season with salt and pepper.

4. Spread the tomato mixture on the mushrooms. Top with cheese. Bake for 20-25 minutes.

- **1 pound** Portobello Mushroom, gill removed and thinly sliced

- 1 14.5-ounce **can** crushed tomatoes

- **1 cup** fat-free parmesan cheese

- **1 cup** fat-free cheddar cheese

- **2 tablespoons** chopped fresh parsley

- **2 tablespoons** chopped fresh basil

- **1 teaspoon** dried oregano

- salt and pepper to taste

- Nonstick Cooking Spray

CALORIES	CARBS	SUGAR	FAT	PROTEIN	SODIUM
105	14.2	1.2	1.3	11.6	393
KCAL	GRAMS	GRAMS	GRAMS	GRAMS	MILLIGRAMS

BAKED GARLIC TOFU

SERVES
4

PREP TIME
10
MINUTES

COOK TIME
40
MINUTES

- 1 14-ounce **block** firm tofu, diced

- 4 **cloves** garlic, minced

- 2 **tablespoons** low-sodium soy sauce

- 1 **tablespoon** cornstarch

- 2 **teaspoons** stevia

- 1 **teaspoon** sriracha sauce

- 1 **teaspoon** onion powder

1. Preheat the oven to 400°F. Bake the tofu for 35-40 minutes until golden. Flipping once.

2. Spray a sauce pan, sauté garlic until fragrant. Add soy sauce, onion powder, stevia and sriracha sauce.

3. Dissolve the cornstarch in a few tablespoons of water. Slowly stir in the cornstarch mixture. Cook until sauce thickens.

CALORIES	CARBS	SUGAR	FAT	PROTEIN	SODIUM
102	6.6	0.3	4.7	8.9	325
KCAL	GRAMS	GRAMS	GRAMS	GRAMS	MILLIGRAMS

Cooking Information Summary

Method: B-Baking   BR-Braising   G-Grilling   PF-Pan Fry   SF-Stir Fry

Recipe Name	Time (min)	Method	No. of Ingredients	No. of condiments/ spice/herbs	Dairy Free?
Beef and Vegetables Stir Fry	25	SF	6	4	Yes
Thai Ground Beef	30	BR	4	7	Yes
Spicy Beef with Bok Choy	35	SF	3	4	Yes
Beef Stuffed Bell Pepper	40	B	7	5	
Salisbury Steak with Mushroom Sauce	40	BR	8	0	Yes
Mexican Beef Skillet	45	BR	5	4	Yes
Indian Beef Curry	50	BR	6	5	
Skinny Enchiladas	55	B	6	2	
Beef Chili	70	BR	4	6	Yes
Cheese-stuffed Meatloaf	80	B	5	0	
Italian Parmesan Meatballs	90	B	4	3	
Cabbage and Beef Bake	95	B	9	0	
Beer Braised Beef	185	BR	3	3	Yes
Sichuan Spicy Beef Stew	135	BR	2	12	Yes
Mongolian Beef Skewer	490	G	1	6	Yes
Chicken and Sugar Snap Pea Stir Fry	25	SF	3	2	Yes
lemon Thyme Chicken	35	BR	3	2	Yes
Pepper stuffed Cajun chicken	35	B	4	1	

Recipe Name	Time (min)	Method	No. of Ingredients	No. of condiments/ spice/herbs	Dairy Free?
Spinach Feta Chicken Roll	35	B	5	3	
Creamy Salsa Chicken	40	B	3	1	
Yogurt Chicken Parmesan	55	B	3	1	
Hungarian Chicken Paprikash	60	BR	5	2	
Rosemary Braised Chicken	60	B	3	2	Yes
Indonesian Coconut Chicken Opor	65	BR	4	7	Yes
Italian Stuffed Chicken Breast	65	B	4	3	
White Bean and Chicken Chili	65	BR	4	6	Yes
Northern Italian Chicken Stew	70	BR	5	5	Yes
Mustard and wine braised chicken	70	BR	3	4	Yes
Yakitori Chicken	490	G	4	3	Yes
Tuna Poke	10	/	2	3	Yes
Broiled Curry Salmon	20	G	1	3	Yes
Portobello Tuna Melt	25	B	7	1	
Buffalo Ranch Salmon	25	B	2	2	Yes
Lemon Glazed Salmon	25	BR	5	2	Yes
Smoked Salmon Scramble	25	SF	4	1	Yes
Tilapia Tomato Alfredo	25	BR	5	2	
Spicy Halibut Parmesan	25	B	3	2	
Asian Salmon Meatballs	30	B	4	2	Yes
Spicy Peanut Salmon Burger	30	B	6	2	

Recipe Name	Time (min)	Method	No. of Ingredients	No. of condiments/ spice/herbs	Dairy Free?
Asian Ginger catfish	35	BR	4	4	Yes
Cheesy Tuna Mini Casserole	40	B	6	1	
Mediterranean White Fish	45	BR	5	5	
Garlic Herb Tuna Steak	50	G	2	2	Yes
Spicy Tuna Cakes	60	B	4	3	Yes
Balsamic Pork tenderloin	25	BR	5	1	Yes
Pork and Broccoli Stir Fry	25	SF	4	3	Yes
Pork Chop in Mushroom Sauce	50	BR	5	1	
Pork Chop in Creamy Onion sauce	50	BR	4	2	
Pork Stroganoff	50	BR	6	6	
Vinegar Mustard Glazed Ham Loaf	100	B	5	3	
Garlic Lemon Scallops	15	BR	4	2	Yes
Scallops in Jalapeno Whisky Cream Sauce	15	BR	4	3	
Lowcountry Shrimps	20	BR	3	2	Yes
Cheesy Onion Scallops	20	BR	5	3	
Shrimp à la Grecque	25	BR	4	3	
Crab Imperial	30	B	6	5	
Steamed Clams in Garlic Wine Sauce	35	BR	3	2	
Mussels in Marinara Sauce	40	BR	5	2	
Creamy Cajun Shrimps	40	B	5	3	
Maryland Crab Cake	75	B	3	4	

Recipe Name	Time (min)	Method	No. of Ingredients	No. of condiments/ spice/herbs	Dairy Free?
Grilled Tomato Basil Marinated Shrimp	135	G	2	5	Yes
Grilled Lemon Ginger Shrimp	135	G	2	4	Yes
Taco Salad	25	SF	6	2	
Asian Lettuce Wrap	35	SF	5	7	Yes
Shrimp Salad Stuffed tomatoes	35	/	4	3	
Sloppy Joe Lettuce Wrap	50	BR	5	3	Yes
Garden Salad with lemon chicken and Feta	60	PF	5	2	
Buffalo Chicken Lettuce Wrap	70	BR	5	1	
Seared Tandoori Tofu	15	PF	1	4	Yes
Italian Portobello Bake	30	B	3	3	
Baked Garlic Tofu	50	B	3	4	Yes

Nutrition Information Summary

Recipe Name	Calories (kCal)	Carbs (g)	Sugar (g)	Fat (g)	Protein (g)	Sodium (mg)
Beef and Vegetables Stir Fry	99	4.6	1.9	2.6	13.4	337
Thai Ground Beef	106	4.1	2.1	3.9	13.0	270
Spicy Beef with Bok Choy	114	5.7	1.6	2.6	13.5	469
Beef Stuffed Bell Pepper	118	7.7	3.6	3.2	15.6	471
Salisbury Steak with Mushroom Sauce	120	5.0	0.9	2.9	17.0	566
Mexican Beef Skillet	102	4.4	1.9	2.7	13.2	339
Indian Beef Curry	113	6.4	2.9	3.3	15.0	316
Skinny Enchiladas	149	7.5	0.6	4.3	19.9	495
Beef Chili	147	14.6	3.7	3.3	15.7	227
Cheese-stuffed Meatloaf	83	3.6	0.5	1.6	13.7	412
Italian Parmesan Meatballs	116	6.7	1.9	3.4	14.7	454
Cabbage and Beef Bake	131	9.0	4.8	3.1	17.6	313
Beer Braised Beef	96	3.6	0.8	2.0	13.0	247
Sichuan Spicy Beef Stew	84	2.4	0.7	2.0	13.0	102
Mongolian Beef Skewer	90	1.8	1.0	2.6	12.3	210
Chicken and Sugar Snap Pea Stir Fry	59	1.7	0.6	0.3	11.5	118
Lemon Thyme Chicken	55	1.0	0.2	0.2	11.3	56
Pepper stuffed Cajun chicken	91	4.0	1.6	0.6	16.3	522
Spinach Feta Chicken Roll	83	2.1	0.8	0.6	15.0	328
Creamy Salsa Chicken	92	5.5	4.0	0.2	12.0	296
Yogurt Chicken Parmesan	88	5.6	1.4	1.2	13.4	463

Recipe Name	Calories (kCal)	Carbs (g)	Sugar (g)	Fat (g)	Protein (g)	Sodium (mg)
Hungarian Chicken Paprikash	72	3.7	1.9	0.4	12.2	80
Rosemary Braised Chicken	81	1.2	0.5	0.3	11.0	57
Indonesian Coconut Chicken Opor	136	9.0	1.1	4.1	15.5	226
Italian Stuffed Chicken Breast	104	5.5	1.7	1.0	16.9	327
White Bean and Chicken Chili	115	12.0	1.7	0.6	15.2	322
Northern Italian Chicken Stew	77	4.8	2.4	0.3	11.9	145
Mustard and wine braised chicken	71	1.6	0.6	0.3	11.4	105
Yakitori Chicken	64	1.1	0.2	0.3	11.6	343
Tuna Poke	91	1.0	0.0	2.4	14.7	310
Broiled Curry Salmon	80	0.9	0.0	0.9	18.2	256
Portobello Tuna Melt	137	14.8	3.7	1.8	17.5	620
Buffalo Ranch Salmon	95	2.6	0.4	1.6	18.4	469
Lemon Glazed Salmon	83	1.8	0.2	0.8	18.7	132
Smoked Salmon Scramble	97	1.4	0.4	3.9	13.1	320
Tilapia Tomato Alfredo	84	5.8	1.8	2.1	11.3	324
Spicy Halibut Parmesan	68	3.8	0.3	0.5	12.5	270
Asian Salmon Meatballs	99	5.6	0.5	2.5	14.2	296
Spicy Peanut Salmon Burger	120	7.0	0.9	3.4	16.1	477
Asian Ginger catfish	123	3.5	1.2	1.0	12.3	518
Cheesy Tuna Mini Casserole	148	12.0	4.2	3.5	18.0	670
Mediterranean White Fish	98	3.8	1.8	1.3	14.8	340
Garlic Herb Tuna Steak	95	1.3	0.2	0.8	19.7	173
Spicy Tuna Cakes	85	4.3	0.1	3.8	8.7	312
Balsamic Pork tenderloin	77	2.7	0.8	1.4	15.0	550
Pork and Broccoli Stir Fry	78	6.0	1.3	1.2	13.0	364
Pork Chop in Mushroom Sauce	107	6.0	0.9	3.1	13.1	521

Recipe Name	Calories (kCal)	Carbs (g)	Sugar (g)	Fat (g)	Protein (g)	Sodium (mg)
Pork Chop in Creamy Onion sauce	95	5.5	2.8	2.4	13.6	153
Pork Stroganoff	93	7.3	2.7	1.5	13.6	448
Vinegar Mustard Glazed Ham Loaf	146	9.6	4.3	4.7	17.3	755
Garlic Lemon Scallops	72	5.2	0.2	0.5	11.7	450
Scallops in Jalapeno Whisky Cream Sauce	96	7.1	1.7	0.9	12.4	623
Lowcountry Shrimps	75	1.2	0.4	1.6	13.5	448
Cheesy Onion Scallops	94	6.0	0.3	0.5	12.1	460
Shrimp à la Grecque	97	4.3	1.7	0.9	14.1	507
Crab Imperial	76	10.8	4.9	0.6	7.4	423
Steamed Clams in Garlic Wine Sauce	168	5.7	0.1	3.6	18.9	111
Mussels in Marinara Sauce	174	8.1	1.3	4.9	16.9	410
Creamy Cajun Shrimps	69	1.2	0.4	1.3	12.7	485
Maryland Crab Cake	69	4.1	0.6	0.7	11.5	346
Grilled Tomato Basil Marinated Shrimp	77	0.9	0.5	2.6	12.2	361
Grilled Lemon Ginger Shrimp	66	1.9	0.3	1.0	12.4	345
Taco Salad	134	7.6	2.7	.2.4	21.8	376
Asian Lettuce Wrap	121	9.0	3.5	4.1	13.0	351
Shrimp Salad Stuffed tomatoes	80	4.5	2.8	1.3	12.9	309
Sloppy Joe Lettuce Wrap	82	3.6	1.6	2.2	12.8	155
Garden Salad with lemon chicken and Feta	111	8.5	3.1	2.9	12.9	475
Buffalo Chicken Lettuce Wrap	92	2.0	1.0	2.1	13.1	285
Seared Tandoori Tofu	95	3.2	0.1	4.2	7.8	239
Italian Portobello Bake	105	14.2	1.2	1.3	11.6	393
Baked Garlic Tofu	102	6.6	0.3	4.7	8.9	325

THANK YOU FOR READING!

After your bariatric surgery, what you eat play a significant role in healing and nourishing your body.

I hope this book has provide you some new inspiration. Thank you again for picking up my book and going through it.

STELLA LAYNE 2017

Made in the USA
Middletown, DE
08 December 2017